I0440195

Total
Bodyweight
Transformation

Discover How to Build Muscle and Burn Fat
With No Gyms, Equipment
Or
Complicated Exercises

RON KNESS

Contents

Disclaimer

This publication is for informational purposes only and is not intended as medical advice. Medical advice should always be obtained from a qualified medical professional for any health conditions or symptoms associated with them.

Every possible effort has been made in preparing and researching this material. We make no warranties with respect to the accuracy, applicability of its contents or any omissions.

See your healthcare professional before starting any diet or exercise program!

Chapter 1. Introduction

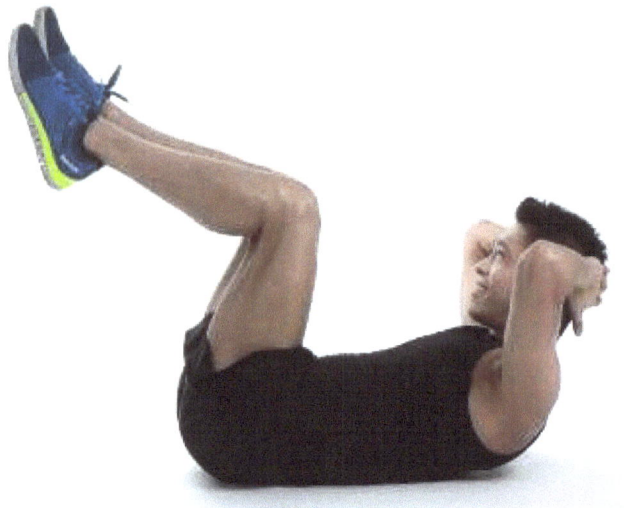

It's so simple… but bodyweight training might well be the one thing you need to start making some major changes in your life.

Not to say that you necessarily *need* to be making changes… But if you're looking for a way to build more muscle, to lose fat, to feel healthier and better about yourself and to be pumped full of energy – bodyweight training can do all that.

And this is true *even if* you have failed to get into shape with other training programs in the past. In fact, bodyweight training is the perfect antidote for anyone who has struggled with regular workouts. Whether you tried running, lifting weights or anything else – bodyweight training presents an answer that is easier, faster and more effective – and that's more likely to help you get the results you're looking for.

Even if you *have* been successful with other programs in the past – bodyweight training can be the perfect addition to your routine and can help you to get even better benefits even more quickly. And it's a different *kind* of fitness and strength you'll enjoy too. You'll be strong but you'll also be perfectly proportioned, more full of energy and even more agile.

Bodyweight training gives you power like a coiled spring!

At this point, the first question you might be asking is: why bodyweight training? What's so different about working out with your own body? Why do people succeed with this type of exercise when all else has failed? Let's take a look at some pretty convincing reasons that bodyweight training is what you need…

The Many Benefits of Bodyweight Training

Practical Benefits

For starters, bodyweight training has a ton of practical benefits that a lot of other types of exercise just can't deliver.

For starters, bodyweight training doesn't require *any* equipment or tools. As we'll see later on, there are some items that can help you to get more from your training and a pull up bar in particular is highly advisable. Nevertheless, though, this still isn't a *requirement* by any stretch and you can get away without one. Even if you do go for a pull up bar, this is something that can fit into your doorframe and that won't set you back more than $5 at the most.

This right away is something that gives bodyweight training a big advantage. This means that you don't have to spend any cash to get started with it and it means that you can do it anywhere. A lot of people like to use bodyweight training when visiting hotels and other places they can stay and you can even do this kind of training when you're camping! You can use a horizontal tree branch for pull-ups!

But this also makes it much easier to get started in your own home. The fact of the matter is that many of us can't afford to invest in expensive gym equipment like bench presses or squat racks and most of us don't have the room anyway!

Then there's the fact that having lots of equipment means it's actually quite a lot of work in order to start training. If you're going to be using dumbbells, barbells, a bench, a kettlebell… this means that you're going to have get all of that equipment out and set it up to use. That might not sound like a big deal but if you live in a small space it can involve quite a lot of work and it can add 10 minutes to your training. Bearing in mind that you need to pack it away again, this can be the difference between a quick, spontaneous workout or not having time to train at all.

With bodyweight training, there's nothing stopping you from getting a quick 5-minute workout in even when you're waiting at the bus stop. And as we'll see, this is a really great way to train as it means you're no longer spending most of your day sedentary and going all-out for just one hour. Using bodyweight training we can be much more tactical and versatile in the way we train and *when* we train.

Physical Benefits

Another thing to consider is the way that bodyweight training can impact on your body. Of course any type of exercise should help you to get fitter, stronger and leaner… that's rather the point!

But what bodyweight does better than any other type of exercise is to help you build a powerful 'strength-to-weight ratio'. This basically means that you can become *very* strong without gaining a lot of extra weight.

At the same time, bodyweight training is very active. The very nature of it means that you're using your whole body when you do that kind of training and that means that your heartrate goes up, you burn more fat and you improve your energy levels.

When you work out at the gym, a lot of the exercise you'll do actually involves lying down! You'll lie down while you perform the bench press for instance and you'll sit down while doing bicep curls a lot of the time. This will get your heartrate up to around 80 – maybe – but press ups are far more active and can get it up to 110 and above.

Better yet, bodyweight training teaches you how to use your whole body to become more agile and quick. Bodyweight training often includes elements of balance, of flexibility and of explosive power – and all these things contribute to improved health and performance across the board.

If you want to be fast, lean, light and powerful – then nothing quite beats bodyweight training.

It's Fun!

Believe it or not, bodyweight training can be a lot of fun. We've already seen that it's much easier, more practical and more active than weights training. But at the same time, you'll find that bodyweight training helps you to learn cool party tricks, skills and abilities that make it so much more worthwhile. If you get really good for instance, then you can start to pull of feats of strength like one-armed pull-ups, clapping press-ups and even handstand press ups. This is incredibly rewarding and gives you an awesome sense of progression.

Bodyweight training is also a lot more versatile than other types of training and it lets you work out in different ways that almost feel like games. You can do bodyweight training outdoors, or you can do it using some kind of ball or other tool to turn it into a sport.

What You Will Learn

As you can see then, bodyweight training has a *ton* of advantages: it's easy, fun, practical, quick, versatile and it's very effective and good for you.

There's a problem though and that's that a lot of people just don't know how to make bodyweight training work for them.

More specifically, a lot of people think that bodyweight training can't offer them enough of a challenge to stimulate real muscle gains or real fat loss. The assumption is that bodyweight training is a kind of 'easy' version of going to the gym and that the results are going to reflect that.

This is far from the reality though. As you'll see, bodyweight training *can* be just as effective for building big, powerful muscles and it can be *very* useful for burning a lot of fat. Some of the best celebrity physiques out there are a direct result of bodyweight training *alone* – you just need to know how to use it properly.

This book is going to teach you everything you need to know about burning fat and building muscle. You'll learn the science behind hypertrophy and you'll learn exactly how you can apply it using your bodyweight – just the same as you would apply it using weights.

You'll learn how to train to trigger growth or to burn the most fat and you'll know the science behind it. What's more, is that you'll learn a ton of exciting exercises and you'll know exactly how to put them together into a training program.

But before we get into all that, we're going to start with a very quick, simple workout that you can do at home. This workout is going to be designed to help you to build muscle quickly and to get into lean shape. Even if you only read this one chapter, you'll find that you have the secret to being in the best shape of your life.

Curious? Then keep reading!

Chapter 2. Why Your Old Workouts Failed

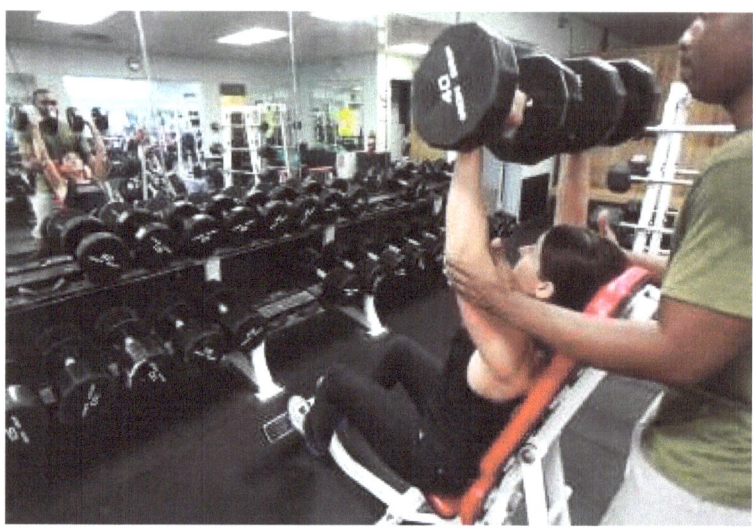

Think about how many people you know who have tried to get into shape and failed. Think about how many of your friends or family members have started new training programs or new weight loss regimes. Either they're trying to build big muscle, or they're interested in losing fat.

Either way, they come to you all excited about their new goals and they show you their program. Often it will involve training five days a week at the gym, perhaps for an hour at a time.

At the same time, this new training program is going to involve eating 500 fewer calories.

How can it possibly fail?

I'll tell you how it fails. In fact, I'll tell you how it fails nearly *every single time*.

The problem isn't that the training program isn't good. The problem is that they don't stick at it. They have this exciting aim and they're all ready to get going with it, but by week two they're already losing motivation.

Something 'important' comes up and they have to take a day out of training. Either that or they just get home from work and they're so tired they have to skip a session…

Then they get a cold and that means another week off.

And their friends are eating out and they're invited, so they head to that and they consume 1,500 calories in one sitting. So far, so bad.

By the end of week three, they're now back at the position they were in *to begin with* and they've made no progress on their diet or their training. This is disheartening and it's also somewhat *embarrassing* when people ask them how their fitness is going.

So they just kind of brush it to one side and then pretend that it never happened. Until the next program comes along that is!

You're probably very familiar with this story and in fact, it's probably a story that you've *lived* yourself a lot of times.

The problem is that these training programs are just too ambitious. Taking on a new training program like this takes an *incredible* amount of dedication and energy, not to mention time.

Think about it: right now you probably feel like you don't have much time in your life. You probably feel rushed off your feet and you probably have very little energy when you get back home in the evenings.

This is why you're currently out of shape. It's not for lack of interest or for lack of trying. If it were easy to get into incredible shape, then you would have done it already! Truth is that life is hard and most of us are struggling just to keep afloat.

Here's a quick newsflash by the way: time isn't the problem.

All of us think that we have a problem with time but this is almost always untrue. We very often think that we don't have time and that's why we don't get everything we want done. But if that's true, then how come you were able to watch that entire boxset of Game of Thrones recently? How come you spent all of last night just lying in front of the TV?

How come you were able to hit snooze three times on your alarm?

The problem isn't time – it's energy. Energy is finite and there's only so much stress and so much work/activity that we can cram into one day before that finite energy begins to run dry.

If you're *already* at your wits end. If you're already exhausted and stressed… then what makes you think that you can add a workout to the end of your day that's an hour long? And what makes you think that you can drive *to* the gym to do your workout? And then back? And then shower?

There are more things about going to the gym that we don't take into account too. For instance, the cost. Then there's the cold weather or hot weather.

And here's one: all that extra washing! If you go to the gym 5 days a week, then you'll be creating five more pairs of dirty underwear and you'll need to wash all those jogging bottoms and tank tops…

You expect to do all this when you *already* have no energy and you also intend to eat fewer calories? Giving yourself *even less* energy?

And you wonder why so many training programs fail?

Chapter 3. The SSE Workout – Super Simple and Effective!

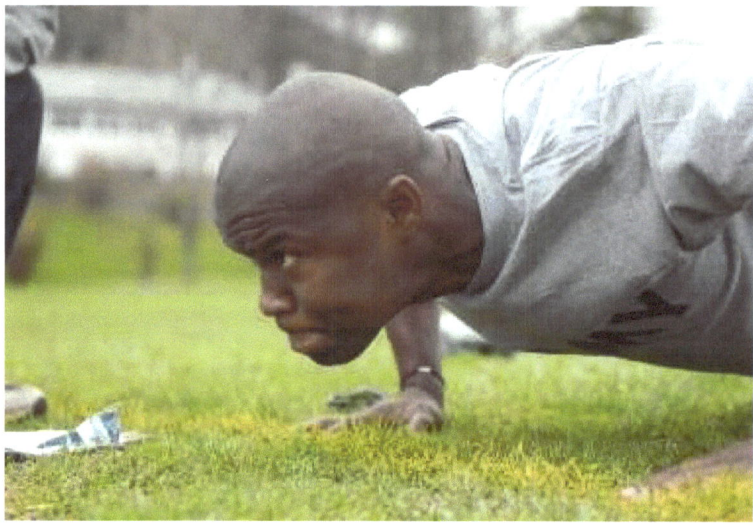

I want to demonstrate the power of bodyweight training to you right away and that's why I'm starting with this simple workout. It's called the 'SSE' workout because it's **S**uper **S**imple and **E**ffective.

This is a workout that addresses *all* of the issues that we saw in the last chapter and then some.

It's a workout that takes 10-15 minutes. All you need is a pull up bar (or a tree branch). And you're going to do it in the morning, before you shower.

The Workout

The workout is a circuit. That means that you'll go through each exercise once and then you're going to start again from the beginning.

You're going to rest for 30 seconds between each completed set and you're going to perform each set of moves for 30 seconds.

The exercises are push-ups, pull-ups and jack in the box.

So the workout looks like this:

- 30 seconds of push-ups

- 30 seconds of pull-ups

- 30 seconds of jack-in-the-box

- 30 seconds of rest

You then repeat it five times.

Make sure that you are doing as many repetitions of each exercise as you can and that you're giving it your all. You also need to ensure that you aren't resting *at all* when you move from one to the next.

It doesn't matter how many push-ups and pull-ups you do. All that matters is that you keep going until the end of the thirty seconds (at least keep trying).

If you can't do regular push-ups, then you can do push-ups on your knees to begin with.

And if you can't do pull-ups (or can't do enough), then you're going to do *assisted* pull-ups.

Assisted pull-ups means that you're going to take a chair and put it underneath the pull up bar. You can now put your feet on that chair and use them to slightly help yourself through each pull up. Don't cheat and just 'stand up' – just give yourself the slightest bit of help with your legs so that you can complete each exercise.

Remember as well that pull-ups are the ones where you use an overhand (pronated) grip. That means that your palms are facing away from you and this way, you'll also be engaging your lats more in the exercise rather than your biceps.

Finally, when performing the jack-in-the-box, you need to squat all the way down and crouch, then you're exploding upward and splaying your arms and legs like a star-fish. It's like a squat combined with a star jump. If you can't do this, then just tuck jumps will be fine to begin with.

That's the whole workout. Like I said, it's simple. But it's also really effective.

And you're going to do it five days a week before you start work.

One more tip: don't do it immediately upon waking. Wait at least 10 minutes as that way your spine won't be soft from sleeping and you'll reduce the chances of injury. This is pretty light stuff though, so you should find you're fine to go into it without a warm up.

Why This Works

So what's so special about this workout?

The first thing is that it has everything you need in it. The workout has three components: push, pull and legs. Each exercise is also compound and that way, you're actually targeting *nearly* every muscle in the body:

- **Push-ups**: Pecs, triceps, shoulders, traps, abs

- **Pull-ups**: Lats, biceps, abs

- **Jack-in-the-Box**: Quads, hamstrings, calves, glutes

You're also going fast and all of these exercises are enough to get your heart rate up. That means if you go as intense as you can, you can easily stand to burn around 150 calories from this alone. At the start of your day that's an *excellent* way to begin and it means you can slip up and eat a KitKat without it mattering as much. By the way, that also adds up to 750 calories extra calories burned by the end of the week…

And because you're training at the start of the day – before breakfast – this counts as 'fasted cardio'. For those who don't know, this basically means you're performing cardiovascular exercise at a point where there is no glucose in your blood. That in turn means that the body will burn *fat* rather than sugar and you'll lose more weight as a result.

Then there's the fact that these moves are actually *quite* tough in terms of the muscle work. You can easily start to notice your biceps, your pecs and your abs strengthen from this alone.

Push-ups are actually *surprisingly* good for your abs. Not only because you're training fast enough to burn calories but because you'll be using your transverse abdominis (the abdominal muscle that wraps around your body like a weight belt) in order to hold your stomach in. This will make your abs look much flatter and it's what's missing from a lot of training programs.

Better yet, this is also *super* convenient. No matter how much of a rush you're in or how tired you are, almost everyone can afford to get up 10 minutes earlier and do 10 minutes of exercise. You need to be strict with yourself here: never go over the 10 minutes. This defies the object and means you'll end up putting it off.

You're doing *just* 10 minutes. But it's enough to build more strength, more energy and more lean muscle mass.

The other big advantage is that you're doing this before your shower. And you can wear the clothes you slept in! Just some underwear will be fine even because you're training in the comfort of your own home. So in a pair of boxer shorts or panties, you can perform your push and pull-ups and then jump straight in the shower.

Now you aren't having an 'extra' shower that takes up time and you don't have any more clothes to wash. This is a ten-minute workout that *really is* only ten minutes long!

This is something that *everyone* can afford to add to their regime therefore and it's enough to help you lose more weight, build more muscle and generally get a lot stronger and fitter.

If you already workout regularly – even if you're an athlete or a bodybuilder – then just adding this little bit of extra training at the start of your day will be enough to help you through patches where you miss workouts and to ensure you get that little bit more exercise throughout the day. Simply put, the SSE workout is the solution to all of your training problems – so add it to your regimen!

Now you have something to start doing right away… so start doing it!

Don't wait until you've read the rest of this book. Don't wait until you've spoken with a personal trainer, **however do speak with your healthcare provider before starting any exercise or nutrition program**.

All that really matters, is that you start doing *something*. You'll learn more as we go through the book but in the meantime just start doing that one thing and start making progress!

Variations

As you get a little more advanced, you might start to find that the 'SSE' workout is a little *too* simplistic. Or maybe you want to adapt it to be a little more 'total body'. Or maybe you just need a change.

In that case, you can do so by simply adding some extra moves to your regime and swapping them in and out:

- Dips (you can do this with two chairs opposite one another)

- Tricep dips

- Chin-ups

- Incline press-ups

Just make sure that you have one compound push movement, one pull and one exercise for the legs!

Chapter 4. How to Build BIG Muscle with Bodyweight Training

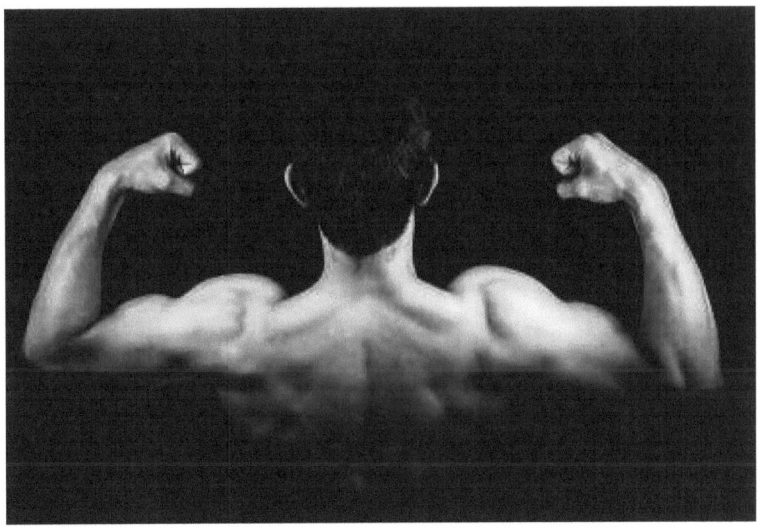

But what if you want to become the next Arnold Schwarzenegger? What if you want to become incredibly bulky and ripped? In that case, you might think that your only option is to start lifting weights but you would be wrong – in fact there are a number of ways you can build big muscle using bodyweight alone and it's probably a lot easier than you suspect.

In this chapter, we're going to be looking at how building muscle works and we're going to look at how you can do it using bodyweight. This is all about theory. Towards the end of the book we'll be looking at the individual bodyweight moves you can use and providing a kind of glossary of exercises for you to dip in and out of. So read this and then apply it to those moves. Although to be honest, you can do most of this with just the regular few bodyweight exercises you probably already know.

So let's take a look at how to build muscle…

The Science of Hypertrophy

Muscle growth in response to training is technically known as 'hypertrophy'. Hypertrophy is what bodybuilding is all about and if you're trying to look big and bulky, it's what you need to be all about as well.

So the question is: how does hypertrophy work? How can you stimulate your body to produce more muscle?

And the answer is that you need to provide the body with *volume*. Volume is what defines the intensity of your training and from a workout perspective, it can come either from increasing the weight or from increasing the number of repetitions. Or both.

This then triggers changes in the muscle that causes it to grow and there is widely believed to be two different mechanisms through which this can occur:

- Sarcoplasmic hypertrophy

- Myofibrillar hypertrophy

Sarcoplasmic Hypertrophy

Sarcoplasmic hypertrophy is the type of hypertrophy that is caused when you increase the number of repetitions. This is the kind of muscle growth that you get when you train with rep-ranges of around 12-15 or even higher. It's also increased when you increase your 'time under tension' which is the amount of time you spend actually straining under the weight (rather than setting it down to rest between sets).

When you increase the number of repetitions you perform and when you hold the weight in position, you are calling on your muscle's endurance. This in turn relies on the amount of fluid and the amount of energy (ATP) stored in the muscle cells – the sarcoplasm.

When you use this kind of training, it means that the muscle is constantly tensed and working. In turn, this causes the blood to 'occlude'. In other words, it gets sent to the muscle and it stays there. This is also what causes us to get the feeling of 'pump' when we're working out. As this happens, you also get a build-up of metabolites – muscle-building products that are found in the blood and that end up flooding the muscles. Metabolites include the likes of testosterone, growth hormone and IGF1. You also get a lot of nutrients in here.

As a result, the muscle responds by growing and specifically by swelling and taking on more water mass. This gives the muscles a bigger, bloated look. They may be quite 'soft' but it's a great way to get big fast and to increase your ability to perform large sets of exercise.

Sarcoplasmic Hypertrophy

Another thing that occurs as you train is that you create tiny tears in the muscle fiber. These are called 'microtears' and they're so small as to not be damaging in any way or that painful (although this can lead to 'DOMS' the next day – delayed onset muscle soreness).

What these microtears *can* do though, is to cause the muscle to appear damaged to the body and that means it needs to get repaired.

When you're resting later on then, the body will use protein from your diet in order to rebuild the muscle and each of those muscle fibers will come back slightly thicker and slightly stronger than before. This increases size *and* strength and the best way to trigger this kind of hypertrophy is by training with heavy weights. This is how 'power lifters' will train and it's how they manage to get very strong lifting a weight only a few times.

What you also need to know about is the different types of muscle fibers. Your muscles have a number of different 'kinds' of muscle fibers that make them up and each has a slightly different role. In general though, we can split these muscle fibers into two categories which are 'fast twitch' and 'slow twitch'. Fast twitch fibers are capable of creating greater acceleration and greater force – and that means that they are the most useful kinds for lifting heavy weights. Your body will use these first when you move heavy weight and once they've become fatigued/torn, it will move on to the slower twitch fibers. Eventually, you don't have enough power to move the weight – but some slow twitch fibers will remain which will mean you're still able to move your arms!

Building Strength

There's something else that occurs here too though and that's that you are also strengthening your 'mind muscle connection'. This is the ability of your brain to actually *use* the muscle you've got in order to exert force and the more you train, the greater that ability becomes.

Each time you contract a muscle, you do so by sending signals from your brain through your central nervous system. When that signal reaches the end of the nerve, acetylcholine is released across the 'neuromuscular junction' and this causes the muscle cells to fire.

As you do this repeatedly, you are actually able to increase the number of nuclei in your muscle cells (called myonuclei) which means that more of your muscle fibers can fire in response to that signal. This *also* contributes to extra muscle growth, because the number of nuclei is directly related to protein synthesis – the ability of the muscles to use the protein in your diet to build muscle!

Making Sense of the Science

That's a lot of science to take on board but don't worry if you don't follow it all.

All you really need to know is that lifting weights creates tears in the muscle fiber and builds up the amount of fluids in the muscle cells and that both these processes contribute to muscle growth and strength increases.

Both these processes also hurt slightly. No matter what anyone tells you (and some people try to deny this), working out to build muscle *should* be uncomfortable.

It's a very specific type of pain and you shouldn't push it too far. But building up lactic acid (which accumulates along with the metabolites) and tearing the muscle both cause the muscle to burn during your training and the next day. Ask any bodybuilder or athlete and they'll say the same thing. 'No pain, no gain'.

Now the trouble we face is going to be trying to get the muscle to grow using only our own bodyweight.

If you're training with weights this is easy. All you have to do is add an extra 10kg to your bar and you've made it more difficult.

But if you're training with your body, then things get significantly harder. Once you can do 100 press-ups, how can you make it more difficult?

Fortunately, there are a number of tricks and methods we can use…

The good news is that your body doesn't *care* whether you're lifting a heavy weight or not. As far as your body is concerned, the amount of force is all that matters. So we can keep the weight the same (our bodies) as long as we increase the amount of force we're using.

Changing the Angle

One way to make training more difficult is simply to change the *angle* of the exercise. This is called 'extending the lever arm' which basically means that we're moving the weight (our body) further away from the point where we're applying force. This then makes the exercise more difficult because the amount of force generated has to be greater.

The easiest way to demonstrate this is by doing a push-up. Get into push-up position as you normally would but now, instead of performing the push-up like that, you're going to move your arms *down* slightly (so that they're level with the bottoms of your pecs) and you're going to turn your hands to face slightly outward.

What you have just done is to extend the lever. You are now lifting *more weight* because your body is hanging over the top and the force needs to travel further along your arm and at an angle. Although the amount of weight hasn't changed, the amount of force *has*. This is called a 'maltese push-up' by the way.

Increasing the Acceleration

As far as your muscle fiber is concerned, acceleration and strength are the same things. In other words, to contract your muscle *quickly* is the exact same thing as to contract your muscle *hard*.

This then means that we can now use something called 'plyometrics' in order to train the same explosive 'fast twitch' muscle fibers that we would with a heavy weight. The perfect example? Clapping push-ups! Simply perform push-ups as normal but launch yourself up into the air as high as you can and clap once or twice before coming back down. In doing this, you are still performing push-ups with the same amount of weight but now you are launching yourself into the air through sheer acceleration. You'll find you'll fatigue a lot more quickly as a result!

How to Double the Weight

Want to quickly double the amount of weight you're using to lift yourself during a pull-up? The very simple solution is to remove one arm from the bar. This way, you are now lifting the same amount of weight but with just one bicep, one lat and one side of your body. The same applies for push-ups, tricep dips and numerous other types of exercise.

At this point you're probably wondering how you ever *get* to the point where you can perform pull-ups with one hand. And the simple answer is to transition gradually! In other words, you can start by putting 70% of your weight on one hand and 30% on the other. This requires you to manipulate the amount of force you exert on each side too and in doing that, you're improving your mind-muscle connection and also your agility and body control! Very cool.

So perform a pull-up leaning slight more to one side, then move more toward the other side on the next rep and continue to alternate like that. This way, you are going to be able to gradually build up the strength to lift yourself entirely on just one side eventually!

Using Intensity Techniques to Build Muscle With Bodyweight Moves

As you can see then, there are plenty of ways you can make bodyweight training hard. Can you do a hand stand push-up with one hand yet? Can you hold planche (arms on the maltese push-up position, legs hovering behind you)? If not, then you haven't exhausted all the possibilities with bodyweight training yet!

The problem is that a lot of people just don't apply these techniques right when doing bodyweight training to try and build muscle. They do 30 push-ups three times and then call it a day for pecs! Either that you they have a weak attempt at a maltese push-up, or at a one handed push-up and then they give up.

But remember: to accomplish the very most growth, you need to increase volume and that means the amount of repetitions *and* the amount of weight.

And you need to find ways to push yourself *past* failure. If you stop before you're forced too, then you won't cause those microtears and you won't trigger that much growth.

This is where we can turn to bodybuilders for inspiration. They will combine a number of different exercises in unique ways in order to push past failure and increase their volume and their time under tension. These techniques are referred to as 'intensity techniques' or the 'Joe Weider principles'.

They include things like drop sets – which involve lowering the amount of weight each time you reach failure and then doing more reps. They also include supersets (switching quickly from one move to the next), giant sets (performing huge combinations of different exercises with no rest in between), burns (performing as much of the movement as they can once their muscles have tired out and given up), rest-pause (stopping halfway through the movement so that they aren't able to rely on momentum to help them through), pre-exhaust (exhausting one muscle group before an exercise so that the other muscles have to work on their own), cheats (cheating through the move so they can do just a couple more reps)… and more!

This is how you need to start thinking about your bodyweight training if you want to trigger maximum muscle growth.

That means that you don't just do 'three sets of ten' all the time. Instead you might use something called a 'mechanical drop set' which means that you make the weight lighter each time you fail but changing your position.

For instance, you could do:

Clapping push-ups to failure → Normal push-ups to failure → Push-ups on your knees to failure

Or:

One handed pull-ups to failure → Two handed pull-ups to failure → Assisted pull-ups to failure

Now you are fatiguing the fast twitch muscle fibers *multiple* times during the movement and you are pushing yourself far past failure. You've increased the weight, the time under tension and more importantly, you should *feel* this start to burn in the muscle.

Really focus on that – listen to your body and try to feel how your muscles are responding. Can you feel the pump and the burn? Are you getting the same kind of workout from this training as you would do by lifting very heavy weights in the gym? If it doesn't feel hard enough, then you need to go back to the drawing board and start making it *harder*!

You can even use 'burns' at the end of these sequences. So once you've done as many pull-ups as you can, you simply hang and perform as much of the movement as you can and *feel* the muscle burning as you do.

Who said that bodyweight workouts had to be easy?

Split for Bodyweight Muscle Building: Push, Pull, Legs

Note that for this kind of intense training, you should avoid training the same muscle group more than once a week. This isn't like the SSE workout because it's too much to do every body part like this every day.

Instead, split your workouts into three separate days:

- Push (push-ups, dips, shoulder press)

- Pull (pull-ups, biceps, chin-ups)

- Legs (squats, lunges, calf raises)

Use multiple exercises that are similar and repeatedly push each muscle group to failure. You can perform PPL once or twice a week and then just make sure to rest well and eat lots of protein during your off days.

Chapter 5. Burn Fat, Build Strength and Improve Your Health

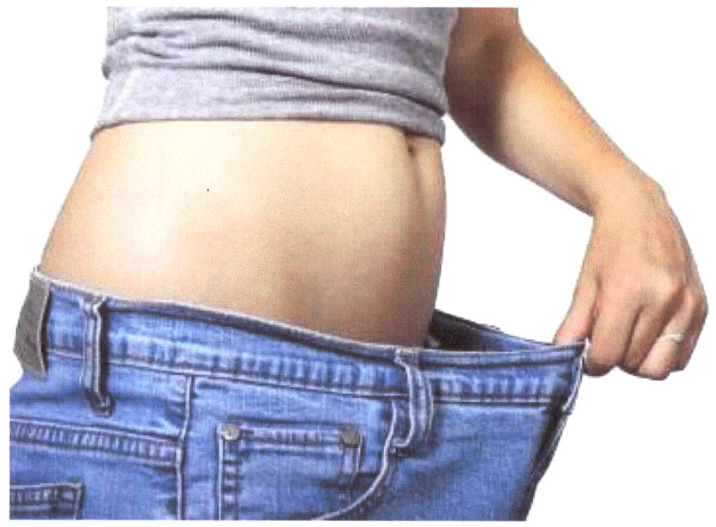

Not everyone reading this book is going to want to build big muscle though and creating intense workout splits certainly isn't for everybody.

A lot of you are going to just want to improve your health, burn some fat and feel a bit stronger. In that case, you can start seeing amazing benefits just simply by using the SSE workout discussed at the start of this book. As you progress though, you may want to make this more challenging for yourself and spend a bit more than 10 minutes in the morning to build some real strength and burn some real fat!

Burning Fat With Bodyweight Training

People who want to burn fat and lose weight will often mistakenly assume that they can't really achieve that using weights or bodyweight training.

This is why you'll find that the majority of weight loss programs tend to revolve around cardio and aerobic exercises such as running, cycling or skipping rope.

Don't get me wrong – this *is* an effective way to burn fat.

It's just that bodyweight training is *better*. Trust me!

There are many reasons for this. The first is that bodyweight training when performed in the right way actually involves more energy than running. That's because you can use *all* of your limbs. Try performing burpees for 30 seconds and then see how you feel! It's just as energetic as running and you're burning just as many calories. And contracting at the same time only makes this even more insanely tough – this is what's known as 'resistance cardio' and it's one of the very best ways to burn fat quickly.

At the same time, performing things like burpees is *also* using a lot of muscle. You'll be using all your leg muscles, your triceps, your pecs, your shoulders… and when you do this, you trigger the release of growth hormone and testosterone. These are *anabolic* hormones that cause you to build muscle *and* burn more fat.

And what's more, is that simply *having* more muscle will also help you to burn more fat. If you have big biceps and pecs, then your body needs to fuel them and that means that you'll burn through lots more calories even while you're sleeping!

There's also the fact that toning muscle at the same time as burning fat leads to a much better physique. A lot of people want to get rid of cellulite for instance. Guess what?

The best way to get rid of cellulite is not to burn fat but rather to build muscle underneath and thereby tone up the flesh and make everything look smoother.

Toning muscle also gives you all the proportions you want. If you're a woman, then type in 'girls who squat' at Google Images. You'll see that women who squat are *famous* for having great buttocks. You can do the exact same thing with tuck jumps but you'll be burning more fat at the same time!

The Workouts

So how do you put this into practice? Fortunately, it's pretty easy.

This time we *do* want to focus on whole body workouts. Doing that will enable us to burn more calories and to trigger the release of more hormones at once. And we're not going to be fatiguing the muscles to the same degree, so there's no reason we can't train the same area a few times in a row.

Circuits lend themselves perfectly to this and now all you're going to do is to make sure that you perform each 'station' with high intensity. That means that you're going to pump out as many repetitions as you can and move straight from one station to the next. Time yourself and try to beat your 'high score' each time you do the workout.

You can also throw in a few cardio moves and then just make sure that the last station gives you a decent amount of time to rest and recover before you start again.

Here's what an example might look like:

- 30 seconds pull-ups

- 30 seconds clapping push-ups

- 30 seconds tricep dips

- 30 seconds tuck jumps

- 30 seconds chin-ups

- 30 seconds jumping lunges

- 30 seconds incline push-ups

- 30 seconds rest

Then just repeat this 5 times for a 20-minute workout! You can replace the moves for things that are harder/easier depending on your ability, just make sure that you are going full throttle (assuming you're in good health of course) and that you hit each muscle group in the body.

You can use this workout 3-5 times a week and you'll find that's more than enough to *really* start toning up.

And if you're looking for something a little more guided that will talk you through the movements, you can always try something like *The Insanity Workout*. They're actually very good.

I wouldn't though. Why? Because you can get tons of free videos on YouTube and free apps that do the *exact* same thing.

HIIT and Tabata

Think the circuit above is too easy? Then let's up the ante a little…

HIIT stands for 'High Intensity Interval Training' and is a *very* popular form of training right now for people looking to lose weight. The basic idea of this kind of training is that you are alternating between periods of extreme exertion and gentle recovery.

So for example, you might sprint for 30 seconds and then jog for 2 minutes and repeat. This works because it allows you to switch between aerobic and anaerobic training. Aerobic training means that you are running at a speed that allows you to burn fat stores by breathing in more oxygen and circulating it. This occurs when you exert yourself at 70% of your maximum heartrate.

Conversely, anaerobic training occurs when you train at 90% of your maximum heartrate. At this point, you are exercising far too quickly in order to burn fat and so you burn sugar in the blood instead. When you do this, it means that you use up all that available sugar and from that point onward your body can *only* use fat stores. It also means that you carry on burning fat throughout the rest of the day as you have lower blood sugar.

There's more to this as well. HIIT allows you to exert yourself more in a shorter timeframe, thereby making the form of exercise much more practical and meaning that you're more likely to squeeze it into a busy schedule and get much more benefit from it.

Of course this can be applied to bodyweight training – which is already more effective than just cardio (it's 'resistance cardio') and which also triggers an anabolic response. This is the *perfect storm* for weight loss.

And it need only take you four minutes a day…

Tabata Protocol

The Tabata protocol is one of the best techniques available for utilizing HIIT and it takes just four minutes too.

The idea is simple:

- 30 seconds of exercise

- 30 seconds of rest

And you repeat this eight times.

Sounds easy but it's absolutely brutal by the end as long as you're training with full intensity. Good examples of things you can do include tuck jumps, push-ups, pull-ups (this is not easy *at all* though) or clapping push-ups.

As you progress, you can also use the Tabata protocol in conjunction with 'active recovery'. That means that instead of resting for thirty seconds, you're now going to hold plank or do sit-ups – some form of 'light' bodyweight training.

Don't try this until you've been doing SSE for a while or regular circuits. When you first try it, only do it for 2 minutes.

This is HARD as nails. But it really does get results.

Training for Strength

If all you're really interested in is improving your strength, then you don't need to do Tabata and you might not want to do intense workouts that trigger maximum hypertrophy either.

In this case, what you can focus on instead is 'progressions'. This means progressing from a relatively easy exercise, all the way up to a much harder one.

You can use full body for this and you might start with a basic workout that lets you hit each body part a few times:

- **Push-Ups – 3 x Failure**

- **Pull-ups – 3 x Failure**

- **Plank – 1 Minute**

- **Sit-Ups – 3 x Failure**

- **Decline Push-ups – 3 x Failure**

- **Tuck Jumps – 3 x 1 Minute**

- **Bodyweight Squats – 3 x 20**

- **Calf Raises – 3 x 20**

Perform this three times a week.

Then, once you start being able do these lots of times, you can begin to increase the challenge. Instead of doing push-ups, you may start doing clapping push-ups – or rocking push-ups (you'll find descriptions of these later). Likewise, you might try to progress from decline push-ups to handstand push-ups with your feet against the wall.

Maybe you move from plank to 'faux planche'.

Then you perform this next step up until you can do all of those things very easily. And from there you make the next step up to something even harder. Now you might do planche, you might do regular handstand push-ups and you might start doing clapping push-ups behind your back.

Training for Health

Finally, you can also use bodyweight training as the perfect tool for improving your overall health. In this case, you can keep your workouts fairly easy. Stick with 'full body' routines but don't worry so much about the progression. Instead, make it a part of your routine and at the same time, try to build in some light stretching and perhaps even some quiet meditation.

For overall health what's really important is just that you *move* and that you actually use your body. Many of us aren't capable of performing a full squat movement with our heels flat on the floor and this is indicative of *severe* flexibility issues. Try getting around that problem by performing body weight squats and going all the way to the ground. Likewise, try to add in some cardio moves like tuck jumps to get the heart beating.

Go at your own pace. At this point, you've learned *how* many of these moves are affecting your body. So all that's left to do is to find the goals you want to shoot for and to gently introduce the right training into your routine.

Chapter 6. The Sticking Point - Biceps

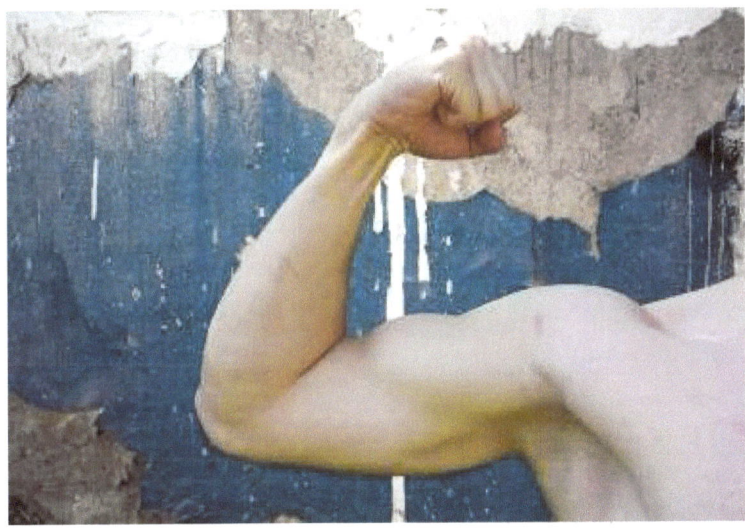

The title of this book promises that you can get into great shape with NO equipment. And yet we *keep* mentioning pull-ups and chin-ups.

That's because training the biceps with zero equipment is actually quite hard. And the same is also true for the lats and pulling movements in general. A pull-up bar – as we said already – can be bought online for $5 and will fit into your doorframe without even needing you to screw it in or drill any holes. There's really *no* reason that you can get one of these.

And if you can't, then there are a few more options. One is to use the underside of a table or desk. Simply lie flat underneath the table, hook your hands under one edge and then perform 'half' pull-ups with your legs on the ground. Or you can even lift the legs up and do pull-ups while in a 'sitting' type position.

Another option is to head outside and grab a tree branch. Or if you're the very dedicated kind, then you can grab onto the doorframe with your finger-tips. It hurts, but it works!

Option number three is to take a towel, tie a knot in one end and trap it in a door (by closing it on it) and then lean backwards holding the towel and to pull yourself up that way.

There are *tons* of options in other words and I really do believe that you should be able to find *something* that works.

But if you really do want to use only your own body, there are still a couple of exercises you can use:

Bicep Exercises With No Need for Equipment

Elbow Curls: This is a strange looking move but is the closest thing we have to pull-ups without the pull-up bar. Basically, you're going to lie on one side, with your legs bent and knees pointing in front of you. You'll also keep one arm trapped underneath those legs and under your body. Now, using that arm, clutch onto your legs with your hand and then *pull* your body towards your legs. As you do, hinge at the elbow and raise your body off the ground.

Curl-Grip Press: Now you'll be in push-up position but with your arms very wide apart (wider than your shoulders) and with your fingers pointing outwards. Lower yourself down slowly and as you do, you should feel the biceps contract through the 'negative' portion of the movement.

Sitting Knee Curl: Sit on a sofa or a chair and tuck your hands under your knees. Now you're going to curl the knees upward towards your body and you're going to use your biceps to do it.

Ankle Curl: Similar, is to sit on the sofa or chair and then to lift one leg up with your foot pointing at the wall on your left or right side. Take the opposite arm and grab the ankle and then curl your own foot upwards towards you in a 'concentration curl' type position. As you do this, push down against your hand with your foot and fight yourself with it.

Dynamic Tension and Dynamic Self Resistance

There are two more methods you can use to train your biceps with your body alone. One option is to use something called 'dynamic tension'. This is the training method that was introduced by Charles Atlas and it's very simple: you just tense the biceps as hard as you can and then move through the bicep curl motion. This way, you're still contracting the muscle, you're still going through the full range of motion and you're still building the mind-muscle connection through the neuromuscular junction. In other words? It's similar to really performing a bicep curl as far as your body is concerned. Just be aware that this method won't be enough to create many microtears and as such, it's not *as* good as using actual resistance.

Another option though is 'dynamic self-resistance'. Here, you are going to curl one arm, while simultaneously using your *other* arm to force it down. Perform a 'hammer curl' motion in front of your own body and just push down on your fist/forearm using the other hand. You can set the resistance yourself and this even allows you to perform a kind of 'drop set'.

Chapter 7. A Glossary of Exercises

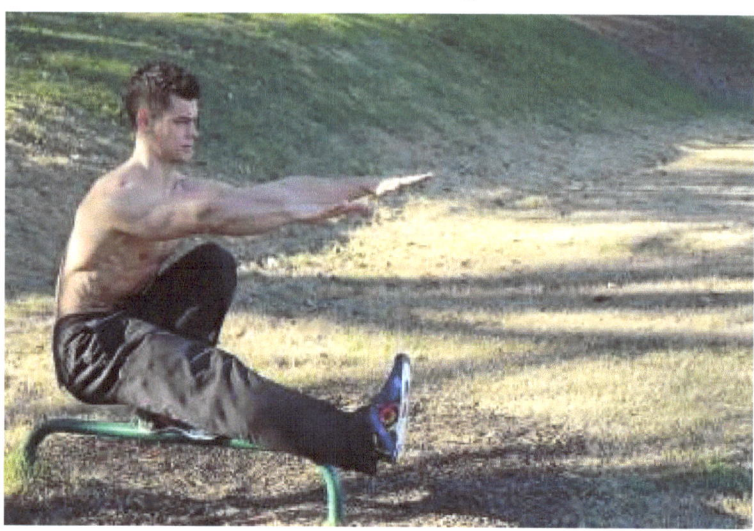

Alright, now you know what you need to do and we've gotten the awkward subject of biceps out the way, it's time to look at some of the actual moves you can use!

Of course there are many more bodyweight exercises and there's nothing to stop you creating your *own* bodyweight moves either. Just use this as a starting point...

Push-Up/Dip/Handstand Variations

Push-ups

You know this one! Lie flat facing the ground, hands shoulder width apart and push your upper body upright.

Clapping Push-Up

Our first variation, just perform push-ups but clap in the air once.

You can also perform:

- Double claps

- Claps behind the back

- Maltese Push-up

We touched on this already: this is a push-up with your hands slightly further down your body and facing outward.

Uneven Push-ups - Push-ups with one hand on a medicine ball or another raised platform. The first step of a set of stairs works great.

Wall Press Aways - For those who can't do push-ups, lean against a wall and push yourself away.

Knee Push-Ups – Push-ups on your knees.

One Handed Push-ups - Like they sound. You can also do them 'Rocky style' and switch from one hand to the next mid-air.

Incline Push-ups - Hands on something higher like a sofa. Makes it a little easier and is useful for drop sets.

Decline Push-ups - Moves the pressure to the shoulders slightly more and the upper pecs.

Rocking Push-ups - Push down more on one side and then more on the other.

Diamond Push-ups - Have your fingers form a diamond shape in the middle of your chest on the ground. This is a good way to focus more on the triceps.

Wide Grip/Narrow Grip - Moves the focus to the outer pecs and the triceps respectively.

Extended Range of Motion Push-ups - Put both hands on something a little raised from the ground so you can do press ups *further* down than you normally would.

Dips - Dips can be performed on any two surfaces of the same height just opposite each other.

Tricep Dips - This is a dip but with your hands behind you on a sofa or another raised platform and feet touching the ground stretched out in front.

Pike Push-up – Push-up with your body pointing down towards the ground. This works the shoulders more once again.

Handstand Push-ups - With or without support!

Sit-up and Lower Back Variations

Superman - Lie on the floor with your arms outstretched and then raise both your hands and feet off the ground. Hold for a second, lower and then repeat.

Salute to the Sun - The same movement but without lifting the legs.

Power Bridge - Lie flat on the ground with your feet on the floor and then raise your body up, propping your upper body up on your shoulders.

Sit-ups - You know this one! Lie flat, then sit yourself up. Make sure to roll your stomach, not fold at the hips. The latter will only work your hip extensors, not your abs!

Crunches - This is even more of a rolling motion. Your abs should 'crunch' before you make it all the way up.

Twisting Sit-ups - Sit up and touch one elbow to the opposite knee (hands behind your head) and then repeat on the other side. Note that your hands should never 'pull' your body up, they're just there to prevent you from cheating. Twisting like this will help you to involve the obliques, which are muscles on either side of your abs.

Leg Raises - Lie flat on the ground and raise your legs slightly to train the lower abs.

Hanging Leg Raises - Hang from a pull up bar and then raise your legs straight up in front of you. This is similar to the 'Captain's Chair'.

Frog Kicks - Hang from the pull up bar then just bring your knees up to your stomach. This is an easier version of hanging leg raises and is ideal for mechanical drop sets targeting the abs!

V Sit-ups - Lie on the ground then raise your upper body with hands outstretched to touch your toes, with legs outstretched.

V Sits - Rest on your hands and hold your legs directly up in front of you.

Bicycle Crunch - Like twisting sit ups except you also 'cycle' your feet as you touch your knees to your hand. Upper body stays raised and never touches the ground.

Pull-up Variations

Pull-ups - Grab the bar with an overhand grip and pull yourself up. Arms should be fairly wide apart.

Chin-ups - The same but with an overhand grip. This targets the biceps more.

Around the Worlds - Use an overhand grip and move your body in a circular motion in front of the bar!

Front Lever - An advanced move: hold the bar and then raise your legs up straight so that your body will become parallel with the ground!

Reverse Push-ups - Here the bar is attached closer to the ground so your legs can be outstretched and touching the floor. Take some of the weight on your heels but pull your upper body up towards the bar. (Like an 'upside down' pull-up.)

'Kipping Pull-ups' - From CrossFit, this involves swinging your legs slightly to build momentum to get you over the bar. It allows you to perform pull-ups in a more 'cardio' like manner.

Assisted Pull-ups - Use anything to assist you while performing pull-ups. At the start of this book, we suggested using a chair!

One Handed Pull-up - You can also use rocking pull-ups to build up to this.

Muscle Ups - If you have a bar with nothing above it, you can perform a pull up and go *past* the bar to then push yourself up with your pecs and shoulders.

Neutral Grip Pull-ups - Pull-ups where you hold onto two parallel bars with palms facing inward toward each other.

Towel Pull-ups - Pull-ups holding onto two ends of a towel draped over something. Great for building grip strength!

Lower Body Variations

Bodyweight Squat - A simple squat using only bodyweight.

Pistol Squat - A one legged squat performed with your heel on the ground and all the way to the floor. You can do a simpler one-legged squat to build up to this.

Sissy Squat - This is a squat where you are on tip toe and you 'lean back' while bending your legs.

Side Squat - Step out to one side and plunge deep into the movement.

Lunge - Step forward and lunge deep on one leg with the other behind you.

Jumping Lunges - Lunge, jump and land in the reverse lunge.

Tuck Jumps - Jump and tuck your knees up to your chest mid-air.

Jack-in-the-Box - Squat all the way down from a ball shape and then jump up into a starfish shape. Star jumps are an easier form of this.

Squat Jumps - A bodyweight squat with a jump on the end.

Calf Raises - Stand on a step or somewhere else so that your heels are hanging over the edge. Raise yourself up with just your calves.

One Legged Calf Raises - The same thing but with just one foot. You may need to use a free hand to support yourself.

Equipment Worth Investing In (And Getting Creative)

Want to take your training further? There is some cool equipment out there that you can use to make your bodyweight workouts more intense.

One great example is to get gymnastic rings. These can hang from any pull up bar and will let you perform ring dips and even the iron cross from home!

Push up stands are also great for doing push-ups through a longer range of motion.

But really, why not get a bit more creative? We've already seen that two chairs can make a dipping station. Three can be used to do some really deep push-ups. Likewise, you can do pull-ups and muscle ups from tree branches or you can hang onto a rope and tie it around a tree.

Or how about taking cans of anything and using them as push-ups stands?

Get inventive – it's part of the fun of bodyweight training!

Chapter 8. Conclusion

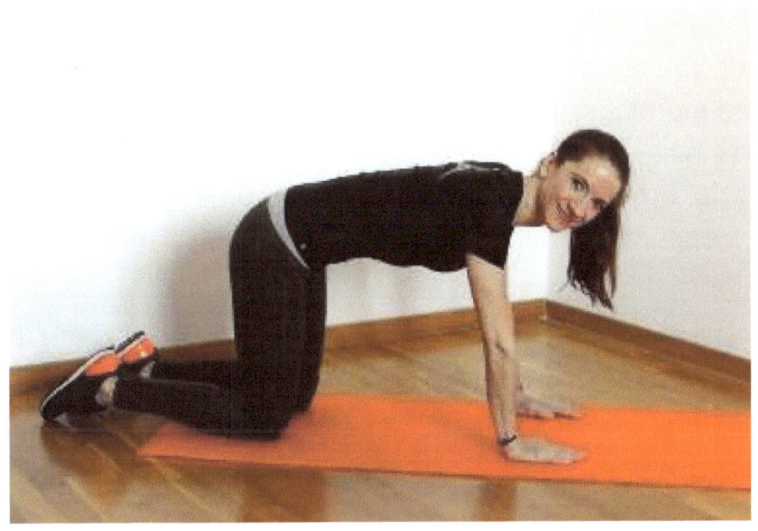

Hopefully at this point you've seen just how powerful bodyweight training can be. This is a way to work out that requires *no* equipment, that's incredibly fun and that you can do anywhere.

It can be used to burn fat, build lots of muscle and increase your overall health. And there's no reason why it can't be just as effective in building size, strength and mass as any training program in the gym. The key is to just understand how it's working and *why* it's working. Using drop sets, super sets, burns and cheats you can get just as much pump during a workout and trigger some real growth (but of course you need to eat plenty of protein to put that into action).

We've also seen how bodyweight training can be used to create *highly* intensive cardio routines and HIIT programs that will burn maximum fat and that will help you burn more calories for days afterward.

Start experimenting with these techniques and see just how much you can get out of your own bodyweight programs.

And if you're not sure where to begin? Just start doing SSE in the mornings. Those ten minutes will help you to build some initial energy, to improve your health and to add muscle. From there, you'll have a base on top of which you can begin really transforming your body with a more intensive regime.

Diet Cheat Sheet

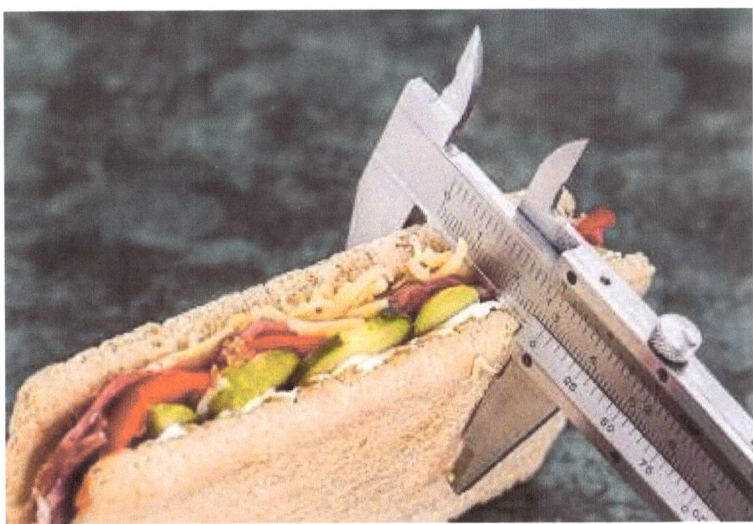

We covered everything you could possibly need to know about bodyweight training in this book. We talked about the benefits, the different methods you could use and more.

But one thing we haven't touched on yet in much detail is the diet. And that would be a rather big omission because as everyone should know – your diet is going to be just as important as your exercise for your body recomposition. If not more so!

A bodyweight training diet is generally very similar to a diet for any other type of training but with a few exceptions. This cheat sheet then will provide you with everything you need to know in a manner that's easily accessible and ready for you to start putting to use!

For Building Muscle

If you want to build the maximum amount of muscle possible from a bodyweight routine, then there is one single golden rule:

Eat 1 gram of protein for every 1 pound of body weight.

While some old-school nutritionists contest this, the fact of the matter is that countless studies have shown this to be optimal for hypertrophy and it's still the practice that every bodybuilder uses.

If you're an ectomorph (find it very hard to put on weight), then you need to eat this along with a high calorie diet with lots of carbs and saturated fats. Carbs are necessary for hypertrophy as they provide the energy necessary to build muscle. Meanwhile, saturated fats provide the body with more protein.

Otherwise, make sure you are providing yourself with optimum nutrition in other ways by getting plenty of micronutrients. These will support muscle mass, strength and more and will help you to prevent illness which can be a big set-back in your training.

To put it simply, the best way to build massive muscle is to *train like a lion*. That means you train HARD but you also rest well and consume lots of protein in the meantime. If you're not training, then you should be either sleeping or

For Strength/Fitness

If your main goal is to become stronger, healthier and fitter though, then you don't necessarily need to eat such vast quantities of protein and the carbs are certainly going to be considered 'additional' too.

Rather, you can actually maintain your current diet while making sure to get plenty of nutrition and to avoid 'empty calories'. This will help you to improve your overall fitness and strength, while at the same time you should try and eat a little more protein. You won't see the same rapid muscle growth, but you will support a general improvement in fitness, health and strength. A surprisingly large number of people fall into this category.

For Burning Fat

For burning fat, there are two schools of thought:

- People who say you should avoid carbs

- People who say that lowering calories is all that matters

Who's right? Both of these groups.

Simple carbs raise the blood sugar and this causes an insulin spike. Insulin is highly anabolic (which is why you still need insulin while bulking and adding muscle) and this can trigger lipogenesis – which means 'fat storage' in plain English.

Another problem with simple carbs is that they're very often the biggest culprits when it comes to empty calories. These are very often things like cake, sweets and processed foods which provide zero goodness while fattening you up. They also encourage cravings.

On the other hand though, simply lowering your carbs isn't enough. And this is especially true if you eat lots of fats to compensate as fats are very high in calories.

To encourage the body to burn more fat, you need to make sure that you consume fewer calories in a day than you burn. This means that you're going to have to burn your fat to fuel even simple things like blinking and breathing as you simply won't have the blood sugar available through your diet.

This doesn't have to be very complicated and hard though. Simply work out your current AMR (active metabolic rate) by using a calculation, or by wearing a fitness tracker. Then work out the calories that are included in your most regular snacks and meals. Keep this number low and then just make sure that you don't go overboard at dinner in the evenings.

Most men burn around 2,500 calories a day, while most women burn around 2,000. What's more, is that most people burn roughly the same as they currently eat in order to maintain an equilibrium. Remove the chips from your dinner and eat fewer snacks and you should find you start losing weight easily.

Quick AMR Calculation

(Your BMR is your Basal Metabolic Rate – how many calories you burn when inactive.)

Men:

BMR = 66 + (6.23 x weight in pounds) + (12.7 x height in inches) – (6.8 x age in years)

Women:

BMR = 655 + (4.35 x weight in pounds) + (4.7 x height in inches) – (4.7 x age in years)

To turn this into your AMR, you then multiply that amount by:

- 1.2 if you're sedentary (little or no exercise)

- 1.375 if you're lightly active (you exercise 1-3 times a week)

- 1.55 if you're moderately active (you exercise or work about average)

- 1.725 if you're very active (you train hard for 6-7 days a week)

- 1.9 if you're highly active (you're a physical laborer or a professional athlete)

Supplements

You can also consider adding the following supplements which will help you get a little more from your training:

Protein Shake: Great for getting extra protein. Look for a low calorie protein shake that is made from whey.

Weight Gainer: A weight gainer is a supplement that helps ectomorphs get both protein *and* carbs in their diet to add mass. This is great for when you're 'training like a lion'.

Creatine: Creatine allows the body to recycle ATP which basically means you can use more energy in the gym. It also improves IQ, is very good for you and can add an inch of muscle by encouraging the muscle cells to store more water.

Fat Burners: Fat burners increase the metabolism. They generally don't work or aren't safe so you can avoid these ones!

Amino Acids: Amino acids come from protein and are used to rebuild muscle. They also perform a lot of other jobs around the body such as enhancing energy and protein synthesis. These may be useful for those looking to add strength.

Resource Sheet

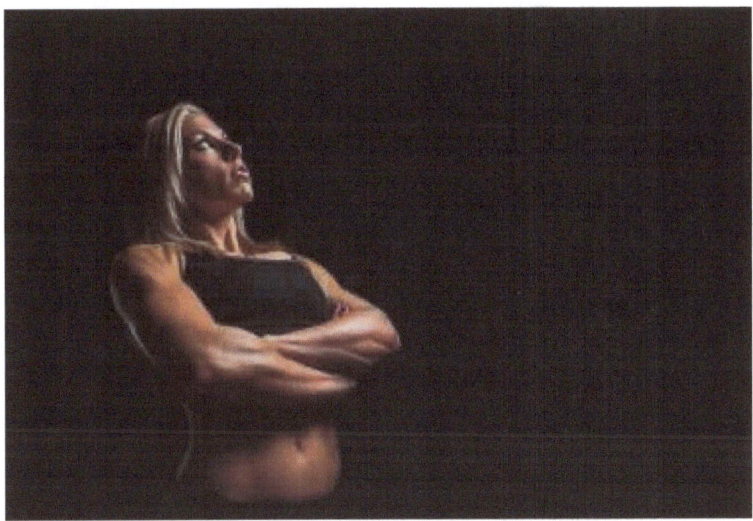

You've read the book and you know how to start transforming your body using no equipment and training anywhere that suits you.

This is the key point to take home: you don't need any equipment and there's nothing stopping you from getting the body you want *right now*. Don't put it off any longer!

But once you *are* already training and seeing those results, you may find that you wish to start pushing your training further. In that case, there are a number of cool gadgets, resources and tips you can use to get more out of your workouts. And you'll find *all* of that right here!

Websites

Bodyweight Fitness Reddit
www.reddit.com/r/bodyweightfitness

The bodyweight fitness community on Reddit does what it says on the tin. Here you'll find a highly active community of people interested in bodyweight fitness. You can check out links, ask questions, get advice and share your progress!

Bodyspace

http://bodyspace.bodybuilding.com/

Bodyspace is another online fitness community. This is aimed predominantly at bodybuilders, but you can find people from all walks of life here. Share your photos, comment on others and track your progress!

Fitloop.co

https://fitloop.co/

Looking for an alternative set of workouts you can use to start training with your own body? Fitloop.co is a great website that provides useful bodyweight programs focussing on strength. There are no tools and you can use the workouts anywhere.

Almost Every Bodyweight Exercise Ever

http://www.thebioneer.com/almost-every-bodyweight-exercise-ever-150-moves/

This massive list of bodyweight exercises includes 150+ moves. This is a great resource if you're looking for some new training inspiration.

Beast Skills

http://www.beastskills.com/

If you were first attracted to bodyweight training because you wanted to be able to do cool moves like one-handed pull-ups, then Beast Skills is the place you need to check out.

Apps

http://fitness.mercola.com/sites/fitness/archive/2013/04/26/bodyweight-workout-apps.aspx

This is a list of apps that provide you with bodyweight training programs on the move!

Tabata Protocol

http://www.tabataprotocol.com/

This website provides you with all the information you need to start using tabata.

Equipment

One of the great things about bodyweight training is that you don't need any equipment. Nevertheless, there are some cool things that can help...

Perfect Push-ups
Use these push up stands to add a 'twist' to your push-ups. Literally! This engages the shoulders and forearms more.

TRX
I'm including this on the list because you likely expect it to be here. These are straps that you can attach to your pull-up bar and which will then allow you to do a range of 'suspension exercises'. They're badly overpriced though, especially when compared with...

Gymnastic Rings
Gymnastic rings cost a fraction of the price of TRX and let you do dips and things like iron cross/neutral grip pull-ups on top of everything else. Ultimately, this is a much better bargain and a much better way to spend your money!

Fitness Trackers

You don't need a fitness tracker but if you're going to get one, then the best options are a Microsoft Band 2 or a top of the range FitBit. In other words, anything with a heartrate monitor which will allow you to more accurately measure your calories burned.

About the Author

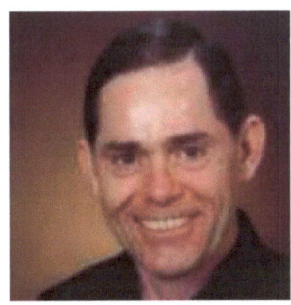 I grew up in Central Minnesota, where my parents owned and operated a fishing resort. Once out of high school I tried a couple of semesters of college, only to quit halfway through the Spring term; I decided at that time that college wasn't for me.

Then I decided to follow my father's previous occupation as an auto mechanic. I graduated from a two-year of vocational training course and worked as a mechanic. While in vocational training, I decided to join the National Guard where I eventually ended up working full-time for 32 years.

So how does all of this relate to writing? In one of my leadership schools, the instructor, who was an English teacher at a juvenile detention center, presented writing to me in a whole new way - a way that started to develop my interest in working with words.

Fast forward about 40 years and I now have over 50 books listed on Amazon for Kindle and CreateSpace.

Besides my own writing, I also ghostwrite ebooks, reports, articles, blogs and do Kindle conversions for my clients on a variety of topics.

Today my wife and I live in Gold Canyon, AZ, where you'll find me happily sitting in my office typing away on my laptop as I work on my next book or ghostwriting project . . . that is if we are not traveling on a cruise ship - our new-found mode of travel.

www.ingramcontent.com/pod-product-compliance
Lightning Source LLC
Chambersburg PA
CBHW050815290526
45792CB00001B/123